Medica

MW00935071

The Key Facts

On Caring For Someone

With Alzheimer's Disease

Everything You Need to Know About

Caring For Someone With Alzheimer's

-Usable Medical Information for the Patient-

By Patrick W. Nee

www.MedicalCenter.com

Published by:

MedicalCenter.com

96 Walter Street/ Suite 200

Boston, MA 02131, USA

Tel: 617-354-7722

www.MedicalCenter.com

manager@medicalcenter.com

Table of Contents

Chapter 1: After the Diagnosis

Now that your family member or friend has received a diagnosis of Alzheimer's disease, it's important to learn as much as you can about the disease and how to care for someone who has it. You may also want to know the right way to share the news with family and friends.

Learning About Alzheimer's

Sometimes, you may feel that you don't know how to care for the person with Alzheimer's. This is a common feeling among caregivers of people with Alzheimer's because each day may bring different challenges. Learning about the disease can help you understand and cope with these challenges. Here is some information about Alzheimer's and ways you can learn more about it.

Alzheimer's disease is an illness of the brain. It causes large numbers of nerve cells in the brain to die. This affects a person's ability to remember things and think clearly. People with Alzheimer's become forgetful and easily confused and may have a hard time concentrating. They may have trouble taking care of themselves and doing basic things like making meals, bathing, and getting dressed.

Alzheimer's varies from person to person. It can progress faster in some people than in others, and not everyone will have the same symptoms. In general, though, Alzheimer's takes many years to develop, becoming increasingly severe over time. As the disease gets worse, people need more help. Eventually, they require total care.

Alzheimer's disease consists of three main stages: mild (sometimes called early-stage), moderate, and severe (sometimes called late-stage). Understanding these stages can help you care for your loved one and plan ahead.

Mild Alzheimer's Disease

In the mild stage of Alzheimer's, people often have some memory loss and small changes in personality. They may have trouble remembering recent events or the names of familiar people or things. They may no longer be able to solve simple math problems or balance a checkbook. People with mild Alzheimer's also slowly lose the ability to plan and organize. For example, they may have trouble making a grocery list and finding items in the store.

Moderate Alzheimer's Disease

In the moderate stage of Alzheimer's, memory loss and confusion become more obvious. People have more trouble organizing, planning, and following instructions. They may need help getting dressed and may start having problems with bladder or bowel control.

People with moderate Alzheimer's may have trouble recognizing family members and friends. They may not know where they are or what day or year it is. They also may begin to wander, so they should not be left alone. Personality changes can become more serious. For example, people may make threats or accuse others of stealing.

Severe Alzheimer's Disease

In the severe stage of Alzheimer's, people usually need help with all of their daily needs. They may not be able to walk or sit up without help. They may not be able to talk and often cannot recognize family members. They may have trouble swallowing and refuse to eat.

Learn More About Alzheimer's Disease

So far, there is no cure for Alzheimer's, but there are treatments that can prevent some symptoms from getting worse for a limited time. Here are some ways you can learn more about Alzheimer's disease.

- Talk with a doctor or other healthcare provider who specializes in Alzheimer's disease.

- Check out books or videos about Alzheimer's from the library.
- Go to educational programs about the disease.
- Find a support group for caregivers, ideally one in which members are taking care of someone who is in the same stage of Alzheimer's as the person you are caring for.

Talking With Family and Friends

When you learn that someone has Alzheimer's disease, you may wonder when and how to tell your family and friends. You may be worried about how others will react to or treat the person. Others often sense that something is wrong before they are told. Alzheimer's disease is hard to keep secret. When the time seems right, be honest with family, friends, and others. Use this as a chance to educate them about Alzheimer's disease. You can share information to help them understand what you and the person with Alzheimer's are going through. You can also tell them what they can do to help.

You can help family and friends understand how to interact with the person who has Alzheimer's.

- Help them realize what the person can still do and how much he or she can still understand.

- Give them suggestions about how to start talking with the person. For example, "Hello George, I'm John. We used to work together."
- Help them avoid correcting the person with Alzheimer's if he or she makes a mistake or forgets something.
- Help them plan fun activities with the person, such as going to family reunions or visiting old friends.

Helping Children Understand Alzheimer's

If the person with Alzheimer's has young children or grandchildren, you can help them understand what is happening. Answer their questions simply and honestly. For example, you might tell a young child, "Grandma has an illness that makes it hard for her to remember things." Know that their feelings of sadness and anger are normal. Comfort them. Tell them they didn't cause the disease.

If the child lives with someone who has Alzheimer's, don't expect him or her to "babysit" the person. Make sure the child has time for his or her own interests and needs, such as playing with friends and going to school activities. Spend time with the child, so he or she doesn't feel that all your attention is on the person with Alzheimer's.

Many younger children will look to you to see how to act around the person with Alzheimer's disease. Show children they can still talk with the person and help them enjoy things. Doing fun things together, like arts and crafts or looking through photo albums, can help both the child and the person with Alzheimer's.

Challenges for Teens

A teenager might find it hard to accept how the person with Alzheimer's has changed. He or she may find the changes upsetting or embarrassing and not want to be around the person. Talk with teenagers about their concerns and feelings. Don't force them to spend time with the person who has Alzheimer's.

Chapter 2: Legal and Financial Issues

Caring for someone with Alzheimer's disease involves planning for the future. This includes getting the person's legal, health and financial affairs in order. It is important to make these arrangements while the person with Alzheimer's can still understand and make important decisions.

Important Documents

Check to see that the person with Alzheimer's has the following documents and that they are up to date.

- **A durable power of attorney for finances** gives someone the power to make legal and financial decisions on behalf of the person with Alzheimer's.

- **A durable power of attorney for health care** gives someone called a trustee the power to make healthcare decisions on behalf of the person with Alzheimer's.

- **A living will** states the person's wishes for end-of-life health care.

- **A do-not-resuscitate form** tells healthcare staff not to perform cardiopulmonary resuscitation

(CPR) if a person's heart stops or if he or she stops breathing.

- **A will** tells how the person wants his or her property and money to be distributed after death.

- **A living trust** tells someone called a trustee how to distribute a person's property and money.

These legal and financial arrangements will help when the person with Alzheimer's disease can no longer make decisions about money or medical care. They can also help prevent serious problems such as financial abuse.

An attorney can help create the right legal documents. Samples of basic health planning documents can be downloaded from State government websites. Area Agency on Aging officials, State legal aid offices, and the State bar association may also provide legal advice or help.

Managing Money

People with Alzheimer's often have problems managing money. As the disease gets worse, a person may try to hide financial problems to protect his or her independence. Or, the person may not realize that he or she is losing the ability to handle money matters. It is important for caregivers to check how well the person with Alzheimer's is managing his or her finances.

In the beginning, people with Alzheimer's disease may be able to perform basic tasks such as paying bills. They may have problems with more complicated tasks, such as balancing a checkbook and making investment decisions. As the disease gets worse, all money management skills decline, with the more complex skills disappearing first.

Possible signs that a person with Alzheimer's is having a hard time with finances include trouble counting change or calculating a tip. You might find unpaid or unopened bills lying around the person's home. You might notice lots of new purchases on a credit card bill or strange new merchandise.

How to Help

One way to help a person with Alzheimer's manage money is to give him or her small amounts of cash to have on hand. Have the credit limit minimized on credit cards or cancel the cards. You can also tell the person that it is important for you to learn about finances, with his or her help. Be respectful and understanding, as many older adults are suspicious of attempts to take over their financial affairs

Beware of Scams

A person with Alzheimer's may become the victim of financial abuse or "scams" by dishonest people. Scams can take many forms, such as get-rich-quick offers and phony home repairs.

Watch for someone borrowing money from the person with Alzheimer's and not paying it back, giving away or selling the person's belongings without permission, or signing or cashing pension or Social Security checks without permission. A scammer might also use ATM or credit cards without permission or force the person to sign over property.

Signs of Possible Abuse

These are other signs that the person with Alzheimer's has become the victim of a scam.

- The person seems afraid or worried when he or she talks about money.
- Sums of money are missing from the person's bank or retirement accounts.
- Signatures on checks or other papers don't look like the person's signature.
- The person's will has been changed without his or her permission.
- The person's home is sold, and he or she did not agree to sell it.

- Things such as clothes or jewelry are missing from the home.
- The person has signed legal papers without knowing what the papers mean.

If you think the person may be a victim of a scam, contact your local police department, state consumer protection office, or Area Agency on Aging office.

Chapter 3: What to do Every Day

Doing things we enjoy gives us pleasure and adds meaning to our lives. People with Alzheimer's disease need to be active and do things they enjoy. However, don't expect too much. It's not easy for them to plan their days and do different tasks. Here are two reasons:

- They may have trouble deciding what to do each day. This could make them fearful and worried, or quiet and withdrawn.
- They may have trouble starting tasks. Remember, the person is not being lazy. He or she might need help organizing the day or doing an activity.

Help the person get started on an activity. Break the activity down into small steps and praise the person for each step he or she completes.

Simple activities often are best, especially when they use current abilities.

Exercise and Physical Activity

Being active and getting exercise helps people with Alzheimer's disease feel better. Exercise helps keep their muscles, joints, and heart in good shape. It also helps people stay at a healthy weight and have regular toilet and sleep habits. You can exercise together to make it more fun. You want someone with Alzheimer's to do as much as possible for himself or herself. At the same time, you also need to make sure that the person is safe when active. Here are some tips for helping the person with Alzheimer's stay active.

- Take a walk together each day. Exercise is good for caregivers, too!
- Make sure the person with Alzheimer's has an ID bracelet with your phone number, if he or she walks alone.
- Check your local TV guide to see if there is a program to help older adults exercise.
- Add music to the exercises, if it helps the person with Alzheimer's. Dance to the music if possible.
- Watch exercise videos/DVDs made for older people. Try exercising together.
- Make sure he or she wears comfortable clothes and shoes that fit well and are made for exercise.
- Make sure the person drinks water or juice after exercise.

Healthy Eating

Eating healthy foods helps us stay well. It's even more important for people with Alzheimer's disease.

Here are tips for healthy eating when a person with Alzheimer's lives with you.

- Buy healthy foods such as vegetables, fruits, and whole-grain products. Be sure to buy foods that the person likes and can eat.
- Buy food that is easy to prepare, such as pre-made salads and single food portions.
- Have someone else make meals if possible.
- Use a service such as Meals on Wheels, which will bring meals right to your home.

Here are tips for healthy eating when a person with early-stage Alzheimer's lives alone.

- Follow the steps above.
- Buy foods that the person doesn't need to cook.
- Call to remind him or her to eat.

In the early stage of Alzheimer's disease, the person's eating habits usually don't change. When changes do occur, living alone may not be safe anymore.

Look for these signs to see if living alone is no longer safe for the person with Alzheimer's.

- The person forgets to eat.
- Food has burned because it was left on the stove.

- The oven isn't turned off.

Plan Enjoyable Activities

Plan activities that the person with Alzheimer's enjoys. He or she can be a part of the activity or just watch. Also, you don't always have to be the "activities director."
Here are things you can do to help the person enjoy an activity.

- Match the activity with what the person with Alzheimer's can do.
- Choose activities that can be fun for everyone.
- Help the person get started.
- Decide if he or she can do the activity alone or needs help.
- Watch to see if the person gets frustrated.
- Make sure he or she feels successful and has fun.
- Let him or her watch, if that is more enjoyable.

The person with Alzheimer's can do different activities each day. This keeps the day interesting and fun. The following sections may give you some ideas.

Household Chores

Doing household chores can boost the person's self-esteem.
When the person helps you, don't forget to say "thank you."
The person could

- wash dishes, set the table, or prepare food
- sweep the floor
- polish shoes
- sort mail and clip coupons
- sort socks and fold laundry
- sort recycling materials or other things.

Cooking and Baking

Cooking and baking can bring the person with Alzheimer's a
lot of joy. He or she might help

- decide on what is needed to prepare the dish
- make the dish
- measure, mix, and pour
- tell someone else how to prepare a recipe
- taste the food
- watch others prepare food.

Children

Being around children also can be fun. It gives the person
with Alzheimer's someone to talk with and may bring back

happy memories. It also can help the person realize how much he or she still can love others.

Here are some things the person might enjoy doing with children.

- Play a simple board game.
- Read stories or books.
- Visit family members who have small children.
- Walk in the park or around schoolyards.
- Go to sports or school events that involve young people.
- Talk about fond memories from childhood.

Music and Dancing

People with Alzheimer's may like music because it brings back happy memories and feelings. Some people feel the rhythm and may want to dance. Others enjoy listening to or talking about their favorite music. Even if the person with Alzheimer's has trouble finding the right words to speak, he or she still may be able to sing songs from the past.

Consider the following musical activities.

- Play CDs, tapes, or records.
- Talk about the music and the singer.
- Ask what he or she was doing when the song was popular.

- Talk about the music and past events.
- Sing or dance to well-known songs.
- Play musical games like "Name That Tune."
- Attend a concert or musical program.

Pets

Many people with Alzheimer's enjoy pets, such as dogs, cats, or birds. Pets may help "bring them to life." Pets also can help people feel more loved and less worried.
Here are some suggested activities with pets.

- Care for, feed, or groom the pet.
- Walk the pet.
- Sit and hold the pet.

Gardening

Gardening is a way to be part of nature. It also may help people remember past days and fun times. Gardening can help the person focus on what he or she still can do.
Here are some suggested gardening activities.

- Take care of indoor or outdoor plants.
- Plant flowers and vegetables.
- Water the plants when needed.
  - Talk about how much the plants are growing.

Chapter 4: Bathing, Dressing, Grooming

At some point, people with Alzheimer's disease will need help with bathing, grooming, and dressing. Because these are private activities, people may not want help. They may feel embarrassed about being naked in front of caregivers. They also may feel angry about not being able to care for themselves.

Bathing

Helping people with Alzheimer's disease take a bath or shower can be one of the hardest things you do. Planning can help make the person's bath time better for both of you. The person with Alzheimer's may be afraid. To reduce these fears, follow the person's lifelong bathing habits, such as doing the bath or shower in the morning or before going to bed. Here are other tips for bathing.

Bathing Safety Tips

- Never leave a confused or frail person alone in the tub or shower.

- Always check the water temperature before he or she gets in the tub or shower.
- Use plastic containers for shampoo or soap to prevent them from breaking.
- Use a hand-held showerhead.
- Place a rubber bath mat and put safety bars in the tub.
- Place a sturdy shower chair in the tub or shower. This will support a person who is unsteady, and it could prevent falls. You can get shower chairs at drug stores and medical supply stores.
- Do not use bath oil. It can make the tub slippery and may cause urinary tract infections.

Preparing for a Bath or Shower

- Get the soap, washcloth, towels, and shampoo ready.
- Be sure the bathroom is warm and well lighted. Play soft music if it helps to relax the person.
- Be matter-of-fact about bathing. Say, "It's time for a bath now." Don't argue about the need for a bath or shower.
- Be gentle and respectful. Tell the person what you are going to do, step-by-step.

- Make sure the water temperature in the bath or shower is comfortable.

During the Bath or Shower

- Allow the person with Alzheimer's to do as much as possible. This protects his or her dignity and helps the person feel more in control.
- Put a towel over the person's shoulders or lap. This helps him or her feel less exposed. Then use a sponge or washcloth to clean under the towel.
- Distract the person by talking about something else if he or she becomes upset.
- Give him or her a washcloth to hold. This makes it less likely that the person will try to hit you.

After a Bath or Shower

- Prevent rashes or infections by patting the person's skin with a towel. Make sure the person is completely dry. Be sure to dry between folds of skin.
- If the person has trouble with incontinence, use a protective ointment, such as Vaseline, around the rectum, vagina, or penis.

- If the person with Alzheimer's has trouble getting in and out of the bathtub, do a sponge bath instead.

Dressing

People with Alzheimer's often need more time to dress. It can be hard for them to choose their clothes. They might wear the wrong clothing for the season. They also might wear colors that don't go together or forget to put on a piece of clothing. Allow the person to dress on his or her own for as long as possible.

Dressing Tips

- Lay out clothes in the order the person should put them on, such as underwear first, then pants, then a shirt, and then a sweater.
- Hand the person one thing at a time or give step-by-step dressing instructions.
- Put away some clothes in another room to reduce the number of choices. Keep only one or two outfits in the closet or dresser.
- Keep the closet locked if needed. This prevents some of the problems people may have while getting dressed.

- Buy three or four sets of the same clothes, if the person wants to wear the same clothing every day.
- Buy loose-fitting, comfortable clothing. Avoid girdles, control-top pantyhose, knee-high nylons, garters, high heels, tight socks, and bras for women. Sports bras are comfortable and provide good support. Short cotton socks and loose cotton underwear are best. Sweat pants and shorts with elastic waistbands are helpful.
- Use Velcro® tape or large zipper pulls for clothing, instead of shoelaces, buttons, or buckles. Try slip-on shoes that won't slide off or shoes with Velcro® straps.

Grooming

For the most part, when people feel good about how they look, they feel better. Helping people with Alzheimer's brush their teeth, shave, or put on makeup often means they can feel more like themselves. Here are some grooming tips.

Mouth Care

Good mouth care helps prevent dental problems such as cavities and gum disease.

- Show the person how to brush his or her teeth. Go step-by-step. For example, pick up the toothpaste, take the top off, put the toothpaste on the toothbrush, and then brush. Remember to let the person do as much as possible.
- Brush your teeth at the same time.
- Help the person clean his or her dentures. Make sure he or she uses the denture cleaning material the right way.
- Ask the person to rinse his or her mouth with water after each meal and use mouthwash once a day.
- Try a long-handled, angled, or electric toothbrush, if you need to brush the person's teeth.
- Take the person to see a dentist. Some dentists specialize in treating people with Alzheimer's. Be sure to follow the dentist's advice about how often to make an appointment.

Other Grooming Tips

- Encourage a woman to wear makeup if she has always used it. If needed, help her put on powder and lipstick. Don't use eye makeup.

- Encourage a man to shave, and help him as needed. Use an electric razor for safety.
- Take the person to the barber or beauty shop. Some barbers or hairstylists may come to your home.
- Keep the person's nails clean and trimmed.

Chapter 5: Managing Medications

People with Alzheimer's disease may take medications to treat the disease itself, behavior changes, and other medical conditions. Caregivers need to know about each medicine the person takes. A doctor or pharmacist can answer questions about medicines.

Questions to Ask

Questions to ask about medicines may include

- Why is this medicine being used?
- What positive effects should I look for, and when?
- How long will the person need to take it?
- How much should he or she take each day?
- When does the person need to take the medicine?
- What are the side effects?
- Can the medicine be crushed and mixed into foods such as applesauce?
- Can I get the medicine in a liquid form?
- Can this medicine cause problems if taken with other medicines?

People with Alzheimer's disease often need help taking medicine. If the person lives alone, you may need to call and remind him or her. A pillbox can keep all the pills in one place. As the disease gets worse, you will need to make sure the person takes the medicine, or you will need to give him or her the medicine yourself.

Medications for Alzheimer's

Currently, four medicines are approved to treat Alzheimer's disease: It's important to understand that none of the four medicines can cure or stop the disease. What they can do, for some people, is help them improve for a while from where they started. Most of the time, these medicines work to slow down certain problems, such as memory loss. Slowing down memory loss can allow many people with Alzheimer's to be more comfortable and independent for a longer time.

The medicines approved to treat Alzheimer's disease are

- Aricept® (donezepil)—for all stages of Alzheimer's
- Exelon® (rivastigmine)—for mild to moderate Alzheimer's
- Razadyne® (galantamine)--for mild to moderate Alzheimer's

- Namenda® (memantine)—for moderate to severe Alzheimer's

If appropriate, the person's doctor may prescribe a medicine to treat behavior problems such as anxiety, depression, and aggression. Medicines to treat these behavior problems should be used only after other strategies have been tried. Talk with the doctor about which medicines are safest and most effective.

Other Medications

Certain medicines, such as sleep aids, anti-anxiety drugs, and antipsychotics (used to treat paranoia, hallucinations, sleeplessness, agitation, and aggression), should be taken cautiously. Someone with Alzheimer's should take these medicines only after the doctor has explained all risks and side effects and after other, safer medicines have been tried. You will need to watch closely for side effects.

People with Alzheimer's should not take anticholinergic drugs, which are medicines used to treat medical problems such as stomach cramps, incontinence, asthma, motion sickness, and muscle spasms. Side effects, such as confusion, can be serious for a person with Alzheimer's. These drugs include Atrovent®, Combivent®, DuoNeb®, and Spiriva®.

Many people with Alzheimer's disease have other medical problems, such as diabetes, high blood pressure, or heart disease. They may take different medicines for these conditions. Make a list of all of the person's medicines to take with you when you visit the doctor.

Chapter 6: Help with Home Care

Most people with Alzheimer's disease are cared for at home by family members. Within families, caregiving is provided most often by wives and husbands, followed by daughters. As Alzheimer's disease gets worse, the person will need more and more care. Because of this, you will need more help. It's okay to seek help whenever you need it. Building a local support system is a key way to get help. This system might include a caregiver support group, the local chapter of the Alzheimer's Association, family, friends, and faith groups. To learn where to get help in your community, contact

- Alzheimer's Disease Education and Referral (ADEAR) Center, 1-800-438-4380 or visit www.nia.nih.gov/alzheimers
- Alzheimer's Association, 1-800-272-3900 or visit www.alz.org

Various professional services can help with everyday care in the home of someone with Alzheimer's disease. Medicare, Medicaid, and other health insurance plans may help pay for these services. Contact Eldercare Locator to find the services you need in your area by calling 1-800-677-1116 or visiting www.eldercare.gov.

Home Health Care Services

Home health care agencies send a home health aide or nurse to your home to help you care for a person with Alzheimer's. They may come for a few hours or stay for 24 hours and are paid by the hour.

Some home health aides are better trained and supervised than others. Ask your doctor or other health care professional about good home health care services in your area. Get as much information as possible about a service before you sign an agreement. Also, ask for and check references

Here are some questions to ask before signing a home health care agreement.

- Is your service licensed and accredited?
- How much do your services cost?
- What is included and not included in your services?
- How many days a week and hours a day will an aide come to my home?
- How do you check the background and experience of your home health aides?
- How do you train your home health aides?
- What types of emergency care can you provide?
- Who do I contact if there is a problem?

Meal Services

Meal services bring hot meals to the person's home or your home. The delivery staff does not feed the person. The person with Alzheimer's disease must qualify for the service based on local guidelines. Some groups do not charge for their services. Others may charge a small fee. For information, call Eldercare Locator at 1-800-677-1116 or go to www.eldercare.gov or Meals on Wheels at 703-548-5558.

Adult Day Care Services

Adult day care services provide a safe environment, activities, and staff who take care of the person with Alzheimer's at their own facility. This provides a much-needed break for you. Many programs provide transportation between the person's home and the facility.

Adult day care services generally charge by the hour. Most insurance plans do not cover these costs. To find adult day care services in your area, contact the National Adult Day Services Association at 1-877-745-1440.

Respite Services

Respite services provide short stays, from a few days to a few weeks, in a nursing home or other place for the person with

Alzheimer's disease. This care allows you to get a break or go on a vacation.

Respite services charge by the number of days or weeks that services are provided. Medicare or Medicaid may cover the cost of up to 5 days in a row of respite care in an inpatient facility. Most private insurance plans do not cover these costs. To find respite services in your community, visit the National Respite Locator Service at www.respitelocator.org.

Geriatric Care Managers

Geriatric care managers visit your home to assess your needs and suggest and arrange home-care services. They charge by the hour. Most insurance plans don't cover these costs. To find a geriatric care manager, contact the National Association of Professional Geriatric Care Managers at 1-520-881-8008.

Mental Health Professionals and Social Workers

Mental health professionals and social workers help you deal with any stress you may be feeling. They help you understand feelings, such as anger, sadness, or feeling out of control. They can also help you make plans for unexpected or sudden events.

Mental health professionals charge by the hour. Medicare, Medicaid, and some private health insurance plans may cover some of these costs. Ask your health insurance plan which mental health counselors and services it covers. Then check with your doctor, local family service agencies, and community mental health agencies for referrals to counselors.

Chapter 7: Safety and Driving Issues

Safety is an important issue in caring for a person with Alzheimer's disease. Even with the best-laid plans, accidents can happen. Checking the safety of your home, keeping the person from wandering and preventing him or her from driving when driving skills decline are some ways you can minimize hazardous situations.

Changes in Home Management Skills

Over time, people with Alzheimer's disease become less able to manage things around the house. For example, they may not remember

- if they turned off the oven or left the water running
- how to use the phone in an emergency
- to stay away from dangerous things around the house, such as certain medicines or household cleaners
- where things are in their own home.

Create a Safe Home Environment

Here are some things you can do in your home environment to help keep the person with Alzheimer's safe.

- Simplify your home. Too much furniture can make it hard to move freely.
- Get rid of clutter, such as piles of newspapers and magazines.
- Have a sturdy handrail on your stairway. Put carpet on stairs or add safety grip strips.
- Put a gate across the stairs if the person has balance problems.

Use Home Safety Devices

As a caregiver, you can do many things to make a house safer for people with Alzheimer's. Add the following to your home if you don't already have them in place.

- smoke and carbon monoxide alarms in or near the kitchen and in all bedrooms
- emergency phone numbers (ambulance, poison control, doctors, hospital, etc.) and your home address near all telephones
- safety knobs on the stove and a shut-off switch
- childproof plugs for unused electrical outlets.

Lock Up or Remove Some Items

Lock up or remove the following from your home.

- all prescription and over-the-counter medicines
- alcohol
- cleaning products, dangerous chemicals such as paint thinner, matches, scissors, knives, etc.
- small throw rugs
- poisonous plants—call the U.S. National Poison Control Hotline at 1-800-222-1222 to find out which houseplants are poisonous
- all guns and other weapons
- gasoline cans and other dangerous items in the garage.

Reduce the Risk of Falls

To reduce the risk of falls, make sure the person has good floor traction for walking or pacing. Good traction lowers the chance that people will slip and fall. Three factors affect traction:

- The kind of floor surface. A smooth or waxed floor of tile, linoleum, or wood may be a problem for the person with Alzheimer's. Think about how you might make the floor less slippery.
- Spills. Watch carefully for spills and clean them up right away.

- Shoes. Buy shoes and slippers with good traction. Look at the bottom of the shoe to check the type of material and tread.

Limit Wandering

Many people with Alzheimer's wander away from their home or caregiver. Knowing how to limit wandering can prevent a person from becoming lost or hurt.

- Make sure the person carries some kind of identification or wears a medical bracelet. If he or she gets lost and cannot communicate clearly, an ID will alert others to his or her identity and medical condition.

- Consider enrolling the person in the Alzheimer's Association's Safe Return program. This program helps find people with Alzheimer's disease who wander off or get lost. Call 1-888-572-8566 for more information.

- Let neighbors know that the person with Alzheimer's tends to wander.

- Keep a recent photograph or video of the person to assist police if the person becomes lost.

- Keep doors locked. Consider a keyed deadbolt, or add another lock placed up high or down low on the door. If the person can open a lock, you may need to get a new latch or lock.

- Install an "announcing system" that chimes when the door opens.

When Driving Skills Decline

A person with mild memory loss may be able to drive safely sometimes. But, he or she may not be able to react quickly when faced with a surprise on the road. This can lead to dangerous results. If the person's reaction time slows, then you need to stop the person from driving.

The person may be able to drive short distances on local streets during the day, but may not be able to drive safely at night or on a freeway. If this is the case, then limit the times and places that the person can drive.

Signs That a Person Should Stop Driving

When the person with Alzheimer's disease can't think clearly and make good decisions, he or she should stop driving. One sign that someone should stop driving is new dents and scratches on the car. Another sign is taking a long time to do a simple errand and not being able to explain why, which may indicate that the person got lost.

Some people with memory problems decide on their own not to drive. Others don't want to stop driving and may deny that they have a problem. As the caregiver, you need to explain why it's important to stop driving. Do this in a caring way. Understand how unhappy the person may be to admit that he or she has reached this new stage.

Tips to Stop Someone from Driving

Here are some ways to stop people with Alzheimer's disease from driving.

- Ask your doctor to tell the person to stop driving. The doctor can write "Do not drive" on a prescription pad and you can show this to the person. Some States require doctors to tell them if a person with Alzheimer's should no longer drive.
- Contact your State Department of Motor Vehicles. Ask about a medical review for a person who may not be able to drive safely. He or she may be asked to take a driving test. The person's license could be taken away.
- Ask family or friends to drive the person.
- Take the person to get a driving test.

- If the person won't stop driving, hide the car keys, move the car, take out the distributor cap, or disconnect the battery.
- Find other ways for the person to travel on his or her own. Transportation services include free or low-cost buses, taxi services, or carpools for older people. Some churches and community groups have volunteers who take seniors wherever they want to go. To find out about transportation services in your area, contact your local Area Agency on Aging or the National Transit Hotline at 1-800-527-8279.

Chapter 8: Taking Care of Yourself

Taking care of yourself — physically and mentally — is one of the most important things you can do as a caregiver. This could mean asking family members and friends to help out, doing things you enjoy, or getting help from a home health care service. Taking these actions can bring you some relief. It also may help keep you from getting ill or depressed.

Ways to Take Care of Yourself

Here are some ways you can take care of yourself.

- Ask for help when you need it.
- Eat healthy foods.
- Join a caregiver's support group.
- Take breaks each day.
- Spend time with friends.
- Keep up with your hobbies and interests.
- Get exercise as often as you can.
- See your doctor on a regular basis.
- Keep your health, legal and financial information up-to-date.

Asking for Help

Everyone needs help at times. However, many caregivers find it hard to ask for help. They may feel they should be able to do everything themselves, or that it's not all right to leave the person in their care with someone else. Or maybe they can't afford to pay someone to watch the person for an hour or two.

Here are some tips about asking for help.

- It's okay to ask for help from family, friends, and others. You don't have to do everything yourself.
- Ask people to help out in specific ways, like making a meal, visiting the person, or taking the person out for a short time.
- Call for help from home health care or adult day care services when needed.
- Use national and local resources to find out how to pay for some of this help.

You may want to join a support group of Alzheimer's disease caregivers. These groups meet in person or online to share experiences and tips and give each other support. Ask your doctor, check online, or contact the local chapter of the Alzheimer's Association.

Coping with Emotions and Stress

Caring for a person with Alzheimer's takes a lot of time and effort. Your job can become even harder when the person gets angry with you, hurts your feelings, or forgets who you are. Sometimes, you may feel discouraged, sad, lonely, frustrated, confused, or angry. These feelings are normal. Here are some things you can say to yourself that might help you feel better.

- I'm doing the best I can.
- What I'm doing would be hard for anyone.
- I'm not perfect, and that's okay.
- I can't control some things that happen.
- Sometimes, I just need to do what works for right now.
- I will try to get help from a counselor if caregiving becomes too much for me.

Some caregivers find that going to a church, temple, or mosque helps them cope with the daily demands placed on them. For others, simply having a sense that larger forces are at work in the world helps them find a sense of balance and peace.

Getting Professional Help

Mental health professionals and social workers help you deal with any stress you may be feeling. They help you understand feelings, such as anger, sadness, or feeling out of control. They can also help you make plans for unexpected or sudden events. Mental health professionals charge by the hour. Medicare, Medicaid, and some private health insurance plans may cover some of these costs. Ask your health insurance plan which mental health counselors and services it covers. Then check with your doctor, local family service agencies, and community mental health agencies for referrals to counselors.

More Tips for Self-Care

Here are other things to keep in mind as you take care of yourself.

- Understand that you may feel powerless and hopeless about what's happening to the person you care for.
- Understand that you may feel a sense of loss and sadness.
- Understand why you've chosen to take care of the person with Alzheimer's disease. Ask yourself if you made this choice out of love, loyalty, a sense of duty, a religious obligation, financial concerns, fear, a habit, or self-punishment.

- Let yourself feel day-to-day "uplifts." These might include good feelings about the person you care for, support from other people, or time spent on your own interests.

Chapter 9: Residential Care

Sometimes you can no longer care for the person with Alzheimer's disease at home. The person may need around-the-clock care. Or, he or she may be incontinent, aggressive, or wander a lot. When that happens, you may want to look for another place for the person to live.

You may feel guilty or upset about this decision, but moving the person to a facility may be the best thing to do. It will give you greater peace of mind knowing that the person is safe and getting good care.

Residential Care Options

Residential care options for people with Alzheimer's include

- continuing care retirement communities
- assisted living facilities
- group homes.
- nursing homes

Continuing Care Retirement Communities (CCRCs)

Continuing Care Retirement Communities (CCRCs)

You might consider moving the person into a continuing care retirement community. This is a home, apartment, or room in a retirement community, where people with Alzheimer's can live and get care. Some of these places are for people who can care for themselves, while others are for people who need care around-the-clock. An advantage is that residents may move from one level of care to another—for example, from more independent living to more supervised care.

Assisted Living Facilities

Assisted living facilities have rooms or apartments. They're for people who can mostly take care of themselves, but may need some help. Some assisted living facilities have special Alzheimer's units. These units have staff who check on and care for people with Alzheimer's disease. You will need to pay for the cost of the room or apartment, and you may need to pay extra for any special care. Some assisted living facilities are part of a larger organization that also offers other levels of care.

Group Homes

A group home is a home for people who can no longer take care of themselves. Four to 10 people who can't care for themselves and two or more staff members live in the home. The staff takes care of the people living there: making meals, helping with grooming and medication, and providing other care. You will need to pay the costs of the person with Alzheimer's living in this kind of home. Remember that these homes may not be inspected or regulated, but may still provide good care.

Check out the home and the staff. Visit at different times of the day and evening to see how the staff takes care of the residents. Also check to see how clean and comfortable the home is. You'll want to look at how the residents get along with one another and with the staff.

Nursing Homes

Nursing homes are for people who can't care for themselves anymore. Some nursing homes have special Alzheimer's disease care units. These units are often in separate sections of the building where staff members have special training to care for people with Alzheimer's. Some units try to make the person feel more like he or she is at home. They provide special activities, meals, and medical care. In most cases, you will have to pay for nursing home care. Some nursing homes accept Medicaid as payment. Also, long-term care insurance may cover some of the nursing home costs. Nursing homes are inspected and regulated by State governments.

Gather information About Facilities

- Talk with your support group members, social worker, doctor, family members, and friends about facilities in your area.
- Make a list of questions to ask about the facility.
- Call to set up a time to visit.

Here are resources that can provide information about facilities.

Centers for Medicare and Medicaid Services (CMS)

CMS has a guide to help older people and their caregivers choose a good nursing home. It describes types of long-term care, questions to ask the nursing home staff, and ways to pay for nursing home care. CMS also offers a service called Nursing Home Compare on its website. This service has information on nursing homes that are Medicare or Medicaid certified. These nursing homes provide skilled nursing care. Please note that there are many other places that provide different levels of health care and help with daily living. Many of these facilities are licensed only at the State level. CMS also has information about the rights of nursing home residents and their caregivers.

Joint Commission

The Joint Commission evaluates nursing homes, home health care providers, hospitals, and assisted living facilities to determine whether or not they meet professional standards of care. Consumers can learn more about the quality of health care facilities through their online service at www.qualitycheck.org.

Other resources include

- **AARP** 1-888-OUR-AARP (1-888-687-2277) www.aarp.org/family/housing
- **Assisted Living Federation of America** 1-703-894-1805 www.alfa.org
- **National Center for Assisted** 1-202-842-4444 www.ncal.org

Visit Facilities and Ask Questions

Visit more than once at different times of the day and evening.

Questions you should ask yourself include

- How does the staff care for the residents?
- Is the staff friendly?
- Does the place feel comfortable?
- How do the people who live there look?
- Do they look clean and well cared for?
- Are mealtimes comfortable?

- Is the facility clean and well maintained?
- Does it smell bad?

Questions to ask the staff include

- What activities are planned for residents?
- How many staff members are at the facility?
- How many staff members are trained to provide medical care if needed?
- How many people in the facility have Alzheimer's?
- Does the facility have a special unit for people with Alzheimer's? If so, what kinds of services does it provide?
- Is there a doctor who checks on residents on a regular basis? How often?

You also may want to ask staff

- What is a typical day like for the person with Alzheimer's?
- Is there a safe place for the person to go outside?
- How do staff members speak to residents—with respect?
- What is included in the fee?
- How does my loved one get to medical appointments?

Other Information to Gather

Talk with other caregivers who have a loved one at the facility. Find out what they think about the place.

Find out about total costs of care. Each facility is different. You want to find out if long-term care insurance, Medicaid, or Medicare will pay for any of the costs. Remember that Medicare only covers nursing home costs for a short time after the person with Alzheimer's disease has been in the hospital for a certain amount of time.

If you're asked to sign a contract, make sure you understand what you are agreeing to.

Chapter 10: Resources for Caregivers

Caregivers of people with Alzheimer's disease can draw on many sources of help for caregiving and financial support. Here are some places that provide general support and advice for Alzheimer's caregivers.

- The Alzheimer's Disease Education and Referral (ADEAR) Center offers information on diagnosis, treatment, patient care, caregiver needs, long-term care, research, and clinical trials related to Alzheimer's. Staff can refer you to local and national resources, or you can search for information on the website. The Center, a service of the National Institute on Aging, can be reached at 1-800-438-4380.

- The Alzheimer's Association offers information, a help line, and support services to people with Alzheimer's and their caregivers. Local chapters across the country offer support groups, including many that help with early-stage Alzheimer's. Call or search online to find support groups in your area: 1-800-272-3900 or visit www.alz.org.

- The Alzheimer's Foundation of America provides information about Alzheimer's caregiving and a list of services for people with Alzheimer's. Services include a toll-free hotline, publications, and other educational materials. Contact the Foundation at 1-866-232-8484 or visit www.alzfdn.org

- The National Institute on Aging Information Center offers free publications about aging in English and Spanish. They can be viewed, printed, and ordered from the Internet. Contact the Center at 1-800-222-2225 or visit www.nia.nih.gov.

Government Health Insurance

Government agencies and private organizations provide health insurance and other kinds of financial support and services for people with Alzheimer's and their caregivers. Medicare is a Federal health insurance program that pays some medical costs for people age 65 and older and for those who have received Social Security Disability Income for 24 months.

- Medicare Part A covers hospital visits after you pay a certain amount and short stays in a nursing home for certain kinds of illnesses.

- **Medicare Part B** helps pay for certain medical services, such as doctor's fees, lab tests, x-rays, and medical equipment.
- **Medicare Part D** covers some prescription drug costs.

For more information, call 1-800-633-4227 or visit www.medicare.gov

Medicaid is a combined Federal-State health insurance program for low-income people and families. This program will pay for nursing home care and sometimes long-term care at home if you meet financial requirements. For more information, visit www.medicaid.gov

Other Government Benefits

Program of All-Inclusive Care for the Elderly (PACE) is a program that combines Medicare and Medicaid benefits. It pays medical, social service, and long-term care costs for frail, low-income people age 55 and older. PACE permits most people who qualify to continue living at home instead of moving to a long-term care facility. The program is available only in certain areas.

Social Security Disability Income is for people younger than age 65 who are disabled according to the Social Security Administration's definition. You must be able to show that the person with Alzheimer's is unable to work, and that his or her condition will last at least a year or is expected to result in death. Visit www.ssa.gov/pgm/disability.htm for details. Social Security also has "compassionate allowances" to help people with early-onset Alzheimer's disease, mixed dementia, frontotemporal dementia/Pick's disease, primary progressive aphasia, and other serious medical conditions get disability benefits more quickly. To find out more, call 1-800-772-1213 or visit www.socialsecurity.gov/compassionateallowances. The State Health Insurance Assistance Program (SHIP) is another resource for caregivers. This is a national program offered in each State that provides free counseling and advice about Medicare coverage and benefits. To contact a SHIP counselor in your State, visit www.medicare.gov/contacts.

Help for Veterans

If the person with Alzheimer's disease is a veteran, he or she may qualify for long-term care provided by the U.S. Department of Veterans Affairs (VA). There could be a waiting list for VA nursing homes. The VA also provides some at-home care. To learn more about VA benefits, call 1-877-222-8387 or visit www.va.gov.

Other Sources of Help

The National Council on Aging, a private group, has a free service called BenefitsCheckUp. This service helps you find Federal and State benefit programs that can help pay for prescription drugs, heating bills, housing, meal programs, and legal and other services. To learn more about BenefitsCheckUp, call 202-479-1200 or visit www.benefitscheckup.org.

Chapter 11: Frequently Asked Questions

1. What is Alzheimer's disease?

Alzheimer's disease is an illness of the brain. It causes large numbers of nerve cells in the brain to die. This affects a person's ability to remember things and think clearly. People with Alzheimer's become forgetful and easily confused and may have a hard time concentrating. They may have trouble taking care of themselves and doing basic things like making meals, bathing, and getting dressed.

Alzheimer's varies from person to person. It can progress faster in some people than in others, and not everyone will have the same symptoms. In general, though, Alzheimer's takes many years to develop, becoming increasingly severe over time. As the disease gets worse, people need more help. Eventually, they require total care.

2. What are the main stages of Alzheimer's disease?

Alzheimer's disease has three stages: early (also called mild), middle (moderate), and late (severe). Understanding these stages can help you care for your loved one and plan ahead.

A person in the early stage of Alzheimer's disease may find it hard to remember things, ask the same questions over and over, lose things, or have trouble handling money and paying bills.

As Alzheimer's disease progresses to the middle stage, memory loss and confusion grow worse, and people may have problems recognizing family and friends. Other symptoms at this stage may include difficulty learning new things and coping with new situations; trouble carrying out tasks that involve multiple steps, like getting dressed; forgetting the names of common things; and wandering away from home.

As Alzheimer's disease becomes more severe, people lose the ability to communicate. They may sleep more, lose weight, and have trouble swallowing. Often they are incontinent—they cannot control their bladder and/or bowels. Eventually, they need total care.

3. How is Alzheimer's disease treated?

Currently, no medication can cure Alzheimer's disease, but four medicines are approved to treat the symptoms of the disease.

- Aricept® (donezepil)—for all stages of Alzheimer's

- Exelon® (rivastigmine)—for mild to moderate Alzheimer's
- Razadyne® (galantamine)--for mild to moderate Alzheimer's
- Namenda® (memantine)—for moderate to severe Alzheimer's

These medications can help slow down memory loss and allow people with Alzheimer's to be more comfortable and independent for a longer time.

If appropriate, the person's doctor may prescribe a medicine to treat behavior problems such as anxiety, depression, and aggression. Medicines to treat these behavior problems should be used only after other strategies have been tried. Talk with the doctor about which medicines are safest and most effective.

4. How can you learn more about Alzheimer's disease?

Here are some ways you can learn more about Alzheimer's disease.

- Talk with a doctor or other healthcare provider who specializes in Alzheimer's disease.
- Check out books or videos about Alzheimer's from the library.

- Go to educational programs about the disease.

5. How can you let family and friends know that someone has been diagnosed with Alzheimer's?

When you learn that someone has Alzheimer's disease, you may wonder when and how to tell your family and friends. You may be worried about how others will react to or treat the person. Others often sense that something is wrong before they are told. Alzheimer's disease is hard to keep secret. When the time seems right, be honest with family, friends, and others. Use this as a chance to educate them about Alzheimer's disease. You can share information to help them understand what you and the person with Alzheimer's are going through. You can also tell them what they can do to help.

6. How can you help children understand Alzheimer's disease?

You can help young children understand Alzheimer's by answering their questions simply and honestly. For example, you might tell a young child, "Grandpa has an illness that makes it hard for him to remember things." Know that their feelings of sadness and anger are normal. Comfort them. Tell them they didn't cause the disease. Show children they can still talk with the person and help them enjoy things. Doing fun things together, like arts and crafts or looking through photo albums, can help both the child and the person with Alzheimer's.

7. What legal and financial documents are important for a person with Alzheimer's to have?

Check to see that the person with Alzheimer's has the following documents and that they are up to date.

- A durable power of attorney for finances gives someone the power to make legal and financial decisions on behalf of the person with Alzheimer's

- A durable power of attorney for health care gives someone called a trustee the power to make healthcare decisions on behalf of the person with Alzheimer's

- A living will states the person's wishes for end-of-life health care.

- A do-not-resuscitate (DNR) form tells healthcare staff not to perform cardiopulmonary resuscitation

(CPR) if a person's heart stops or if he or she stops breathing.

- A will tells how the person wants his or her property and money to be distributed after death.

- A living trust tells someone called a trustee how to distribute a person's property and money.

These legal and financial arrangements will help when the person with Alzheimer's disease can no longer make decisions about money or medical care. They can also help prevent serious problems such as financial abuse. An attorney can help create the right legal documents. Samples of basic health planning documents can be downloaded from state government websites. Area Agency on Aging officials, state legal aid offices, and the state bar association may also provide legal advice or help.

8. What everyday activities might interest a person with Alzheimer's?

Plan activities that the person with Alzheimer's enjoys. He or she can be a part of the activity or just watch. Also, you don't always have to be the "activities director." Adult day care services provide a safe environment, activities, and staff who take care of the person with Alzheimer's at their own facility. For information on adult day care services that might help you, contact the Eldercare Locator at 1-800-677-1116 or visit their website at www.eldercare.gov. Here are things you can do to help the person enjoy an activity.

- Match the activity with what the person with Alzheimer's can do.
- Choose activities that can be fun for everyone.
- Help the person get started.
- Decide if he or she can do the activity alone or needs help.
- Watch to see if the person gets frustrated.
- Make sure he or she feels successful and has fun.
- Let him or her watch, if that is more enjoyable.

The person with Alzheimer's can do different activities each day. These could include

- household chores such as washing dishes, setting the table, or preparing food
- cooking and baking such as mixing, measuring and pouring or tasting the food
- interacting with children by reading stories, playing board games, or sharing memories from childhood
- music and dancing, including playing CDs and tapes or singing or dancing to well-known tunes

- interacting with pets, including caring for, feeding and grooming them
- gardening, including watering plants, planting flowers and vegetables and talking about how the plants are growing

9. How can you help a person with Alzheimer's stay physically active?

Being active and getting exercise helps people with Alzheimer's disease feel better. Exercise helps keep their muscles, joints, and heart in good shape. It also helps people stay at a healthy weight and have regular toilet and sleep habits. You can exercise together to make it more fun.

Here are some tips for helping the person with Alzheimer's stay active.

- Take a walk together each day. Exercise is good for caregivers, too!
- Make sure the person with Alzheimer's has an ID bracelet with your phone number, if he or she walks alone.
- Check your local TV guide to see if there is a program to help older adults exercise.
- Add music to the exercises, if it helps the person with Alzheimer's. Dance to the music if possible.

- Watch exercise videos/DVDs made for older people. Try exercising together.
- Make sure he or she wears comfortable clothes and shoes that fit well and are made for exercise.
- Make sure the person drinks water or juice after exercise.

10. What are ways to make sure that a person with Alzheimer's eats properly?

Eating healthy foods helps us stay well. It's even more important for people with Alzheimer's disease. Here are tips for healthy eating when a person with Alzheimer's lives with you.

- Buy healthy foods such as vegetables, fruits, and whole-grain products. Be sure to buy foods that the person likes and can eat.
- Buy food that is easy to prepare, such as pre-made salads and single food portions.
- Have someone else make meals if possible.
- Use a service such as Meals on Wheels, which will bring meals right to your home. For more information, check your local phone book, or contact the Meals on Wheels organization at 703-548-5558 or visit the website at www.mowaa.org.

Here are tips for healthy eating when a person with early-stage Alzheimer's lives alone.

- Follow the steps above
- Buy foods that the person doesn't need to cook.
- Call to remind him or her to eat.

In the early stage of Alzheimer's disease, the person's eating habits usually don't change. When changes do occur, living alone may not be safe anymore.

Look for these signs to see if living alone is no longer safe for the person with Alzheimer's.

- The person forgets to eat.
- Food has burned because it was left on the stove.
- The oven isn't turned off.

11. How can you help a person with Alzheimer's get dressed?

People with Alzheimer's disease often need more time to dress. It can be hard for them to choose their clothes. They might wear the wrong clothing for the season. They also might wear colors that don't go together or forget to put on a piece of clothing. Allow the person to dress on his or her own for as long as possible.

Here are some tips for helping a person with Alzheimer's to get dressed.

- Lay out clothes in the order the person should put them on, such as underwear first, then pants, then a shirt, and then a sweater.
- Hand the person one thing at a time or give step-by-step dressing instructions.
- Put away some clothes in another room to reduce the number of choices. Keep only one or two outfits in the closet or dresser.
- Keep the closet locked if needed. This prevents some of the problems people may have while getting dressed.
- Buy three or four sets of the same clothes, if the person wants to wear the same clothing every day.
- Buy loose-fitting, comfortable clothing. Avoid girdles, control-top pantyhose, knee-high nylons, garters, high heels, tight socks, and bras for women. Sports bras are comfortable and provide good support. Short cotton socks and loose cotton underwear are best. Sweat pants and shorts with elastic waistbands are helpful.
- Use Velcro® tape or large zipper pulls for clothing, instead of shoelaces, buttons, or buckles. Try slip-on shoes that won't slide off or shoes with Velcro® straps.

12. How should a caregiver handle bathing a person with Alzheimer's?

Helping people with Alzheimer's disease take a bath or shower can be one of the hardest things you do. Planning can help make the person's bath time better for both of you. The person with Alzheimer's may be afraid. To reduce these fears, follow the person's lifelong bathing habits, such as doing the bath or shower in the morning or before going to bed. Here are other tips for bathing.

Safety Tips:

- Never leave a confused or frail person alone in the tub or shower.
- Always check the water temperature before he or she gets in the tub or shower.
- Use plastic containers for shampoo or soap to prevent them from breaking.
- Use a hand-held showerhead.
- Use a rubber bath mat and put safety bars in the tub.
- Use a sturdy shower chair in the tub or shower. This will support a person who is unsteady, and it could prevent falls. You can get shower chairs at drug stores and medical supply stores.

- Don't use bath oil. It can make the tub slippery and may cause urinary tract infections.

Before a Bath or Shower:

- Get the soap, washcloth, towels, and shampoo ready.
- Make sure the bathroom is warm and well lighted. Play soft music if it helps to relax the person.
- Be matter-of-fact about bathing. Say, "It's time for a bath now." Don't argue about the need for a bath or shower.
- Be gentle and respectful. Tell the person what you are going to do, step-by-step.
- Make sure the water temperature in the bath or shower is comfortable.

During the Bath or Shower:

- Allow the person with Alzheimer's to do as much as possible. This protects his or her dignity and helps the person feel more in control.
- Put a towel over the person's shoulders or lap. This helps him or her feel less exposed. Then use a sponge or washcloth to clean under the towel.
- Distract the person by talking about something else if he or she becomes upset.

- Give him or her a washcloth to hold. This makes it less likely that the person will try to hit you.

After a Bath or Shower:

- Prevent rashes or infections by patting the person's skin with a towel. Make sure the person is completely dry. Be sure to dry between folds of skin.

- If the person has trouble with incontinence, use a protective ointment, such as Vaseline, around the rectum, vagina, or penis.

- If the person with Alzheimer's has trouble getting in and out of the bathtub, do a sponge bath instead.

-

13. What steps should a caregiver take when the person with Alzheimer's becomes incontinent?

As Alzheimer's disease progresses, many people begin to experience incontinence, the inability to control the bladder and/or bowels. Sometimes incontinence is due to an illness or other cause that can be treated, so be sure to talk with the person's doctor.

Have a routine for taking the person to the bathroom. For example, take him or her to the bathroom every 2 to 3 hours during the day. Don't wait for them to ask. Watch for signs that they may have to go to the bathroom, such as restlessness or pulling at clothes. Respond quickly. Use a stable toilet seat at a good height.

Be understanding when accidents occur. Stay calm and reassure the person if he or she is upset. Try to keep track of when accidents happen to help plan ways to avoid them. To help prevent nighttime accidents, limit fluids in the evening. Use adult disposable briefs, bed protectors, and waterproof mattress covers if necessary.

If you are going to be out, plan ahead. Know where restrooms are located and have the person wear simple, easy-to-remove clothing. Bring an extra set of clothing along in case of an accident.

14. How can a caregiver create a safe home environment for someone with Alzheimer's?

Do the following to keep the person with AD safe.

- Simplify your home. Too much furniture can make it hard to move freely.
- Get rid of clutter, such as piles of newspapers and magazines.
- Have a sturdy handrail on your stairway. Put carpet on stairs or add safety grip strips.
- Remove small throw rugs.

- Put a gate across the stairs if the person has balance problems.
- Make sure the person with AD has good floor traction for walking or pacing. Good traction lowers the chance that people will slip and fall.

Three factors affect traction:

- The type of floor surface. A smooth or waxed floor of tile, linoleum, or wood may be a problem for the person with AD. Think about how you might make the floor less slippery.
- Spills. Watch carefully for spills and clean them up right away.
- Shoes. Buy shoes and slippers with good traction. Look at the bottom of the shoe to check the type of material and tread.

Add the following to your home if you don't already have them in place.

- smoke and carbon monoxide alarms in or near the kitchen and in all bedrooms
- emergency phone numbers (ambulance, poison control, doctors, hospital, etc.) and your home address near all telephones
- safety knobs on the stove and a shut-off switch
- childproof plugs for unused electrical outlets

<u>Lock up or remove the following from your home.</u>

- all prescription and over-the-counter medicines
- alcohol
- cleaning products, dangerous chemicals such as paint thinner, matches, etc.
- poisonous plants—contact the National Poison Control Center at 1-800-222-1222 or www.poison.org to find out which houseplants are poisonous
- all guns and other weapons, scissors, and knives
- gasoline cans and other dangerous items in the garage.

15. If the person with Alzheimer's wanders, what can a caregiver do?

Some people with Alzheimer's may wander away from their home or caregiver. Knowing how to limit wandering can prevent a person from becoming lost or hurt.

- Make sure the person carries some kind of identification or wears a medical bracelet. If he or she gets lost and cannot communicate clearly, an ID will alert others to his or her identity and medical condition.

- Consider enrolling the person in the Alzheimer's Association's Safe Return program. This program helps find people with Alzheimer's disease who wander off or get lost. Call 1-888-572-8566 for more information.
- Let neighbors know that the person with Alzheimer's tends to wander.
- Keep a recent photograph or video of the person to assist police if the person becomes lost.
- Keep doors locked. Consider a keyed deadbolt, or add another lock placed up high or down low on the door. If the person can open a lock, you may need to get a new latch or lock.
- Install an "announcing system" that chimes when the door opens.

16. What should you do when the person with Alzheimer's is no longer competent to drive?

When the person with Alzheimer's disease can't think clearly and make good decisions, he or she should stop driving. But the person may not want to stop or even think there is a problem. As the caregiver, you need to explain why it's important to stop driving. Understand how unhappy the person may be.

A person with mild memory loss may be able to drive safely sometimes. For example, he or she may be able to drive short distances on local streets during the day but may not be able to drive safely at night or on a freeway. If this is the case, then limit the times and places that the person can drive. One sign that someone should stop driving is new dents and scratches on the car. Another sign is taking a long time to do a simple errand and not being able to explain why, which may indicate that the person got lost.

A variety of options are available to stop someone from driving. The caregiver can ask for a doctor's help, ask family or friends to drive the person, obtain an evaluation from the Department of Motor Vehicles, hide the car keys, hide or even disable the car, or use a combination of these approaches to ensure that the person stops driving. Safety must be the first priority.

17. What kinds of residential care options are there for people with Alzheimer's?

Residential care options for people with Alzheimer's include

- assisted living facilities
- nursing homes
- group homes
- continuing care retirement communities.

Assisted living facilities are available in large, apartment-like buildings or in smaller "board and care" homes. They are for people who can mostly take care of themselves but need some help. Some assisted living facilities and nursing homes have special units for people with Alzheimer's or other types of dementia. These units are often in separate sections of the building, and staff members have special training.

Nursing homes provide 24-hour services and supervision. They are for people who cannot care for themselves anymore. They provide medical care and rehabilitation as well as meals and personal care for residents who need help with many everyday activities.

A group home is a home for people who can no longer take care of themselves. Four to 10 people who can't care for themselves and two or more staff members live in the home. The staff takes care of the people living there: making meals, helping with grooming and medication, and providing other care. You will need to pay the costs of the person with Alzheimer's living in this kind of home. Remember that these homes may not be inspected or regulated, but may still provide good care.

A continuing care retirement community (CCRC) is a home, apartment, or room in a retirement community, where people with Alzheimer's can live and get care. Some of these places are for people who can care for themselves, while others are for people who need care around-the-clock. An advantage is that residents may move from one level of care to another—for example, from more independent living to more supervised care.

18. How can you find out about residential care facilities in your area?

To find out about residential care facilities in your area, talk with your support group members, social worker, doctor, family members, and friends. Also, check the following resources.

Centers for Medicare and Medicaid Services (CMS) 1-800-MEDICARE (1-800-633-4227)

CMS has a guide to help older people and their caregivers choose a good nursing home. It describes types of long-term care, questions to ask the nursing home staff, and ways to pay for nursing home care. CMS also offers a service called Nursing Home Compare on its website. This service has information on nursing homes that are Medicare or Medicaid certified. These nursing homes provide skilled nursing care. Please note that there are many other places that provide different levels of health care and help with daily living. Many of these facilities are licensed only at the State level.

CMS also has information about the rights of nursing home residents and their caregivers.

Joint Commission 1-630-792-5000

The Joint Commission evaluates nursing homes, home health care providers, hospitals, and assisted living facilities to determine whether or not they meet professional standards of care. Consumers can learn more about the quality of health care facilities through their online service at www.qualitycheck.org.

Other resources include

- AARP 1-888-OUR-AARP (1-888-687-2277) www.aarp.org/family/housing
- Assisted Living Federation of America 1-703-894-1805 www.alfa.org
- National Center for Assisted Living 1-202-842-4444 www.ncal.org

19. What types of services are available to help at-home caregivers of people with Alzheimer's?

As Alzheimer's disease gets worse, you will need more help to care for the person. It's okay to seek help whenever you need it. Several kinds of help are available.

- Home health care agencies send a home health aide or nurse to your home to help you care for a person with Alzheimer's. They may come for a few hours or stay for 24 hours and are paid by the hour.

- Meal services bring hot meals to the person's home or your home. The delivery staff does not feed the person. Some groups do not charge for their services. Others may charge a small fee.

- Adult day care services provide a safe environment, activities, and staff who take care of the person with Alzheimer's at their own facility. Many programs provide transportation between the person's home and the facility.

- Geriatric care managers visit your home to assess your needs and suggest and arrange home-care services. They charge by the hour. Most insurance plans don't cover these costs.

20. What organizations can provide help with caregiving services?

To learn where to get help in your community, contact

- The Alzheimer's Disease Education and Referral (ADEAR) Center, 1-800-438-4380 or www.nia.nih.gov/alzheimers

- The Alzheimer's Association, 1-800-272-3900 or www.alz.org

- the Eldercare Locator, 1-800-677-1116 or www.eldercare.gov
- You can also contact your local area agency on aging.

21. What federal and state programs provide financial support and services for Alzheimer's caregivers?

Federal and state program that can provide financial support include

- Medicare
- Medicaid
- Program of All-Inclusive Care for the Elderly (PACE)
- Social Security Disability Income (SSI)
- State Health Insurance Assistance Program (SHIP)
- U.S. Department of Veterans Affairs (VA).

Medicare is a Federal health insurance program that pays some medical costs for people age 65 and older and for those who have received Social Security Disability Income for 24 months. Learn more at www.medicare.gov or call 1-800-633-4227 (TTY: 877-486-2048).

Medicaid is a combined Federal-State health insurance program for low-income people and families. This program will pay for nursing home care and sometimes long-term care at home if you meet financial requirements. For more information, call 1-800-772-1213 or visit www.medicaid.gov.

The Program of All-Inclusive Care for the Elderly (PACE) is a program that combines Medicare and Medicaid benefits. It pays medical, social service, and long-term care costs for frail, low-income people age 55 and older. To find out more, call 1-800-772-1213 or visit PACE.

Social Security Disability Income (SSI) is for people younger than age 65 who are disabled according to the Social Security Administration's definition. Visit www.ssa.gov/pgm/disability.htm for details.

Social Security also has "compassionate allowances" to help people with early-onset Alzheimer's disease, To find out more, call 1-800-772-1213 or visit www.socialsecurity.gov/compassionateallowances

The State Health Insurance Assistance Program (SHIP) is another resource for Alzheimer's caregivers that provides free counseling and advice about Medicare coverage and benefits. To contact a SHIP counselor in your State, visit www.medicare.gov/contacts.

If the person with Alzheimer's disease is a veteran, he or she may qualify for long-term care provided by the U.S. Department of Veterans Affairs (VA). To learn more about VA benefits, call 1-877-222-8387 or see www.va.gov.

22. How can caregivers make sure they take care of themselves?

Taking care of yourself — physically and mentally — is one of the most important things you can do as a caregiver. This could mean asking family members and friends to help out, doing things you enjoy, or getting help from a home health care service. Taking these actions can bring you some relief. It also may help keep you from getting ill or depressed.

Here are some ways you can take care of yourself.

- Ask for help when you need it.
- Eat healthy foods.
- Join a caregiver's support group.
- Take breaks each day.
- Spend time with friends.
- Keep up with your hobbies and interests.
- Get exercise as often as you can.
- See your doctor on a regular basis.
- Keep your health, legal and financial information up-to-date.

23. What kinds of services are available to help caregivers take care of themselves?

Building a local support system is a key way to get help. This system might include a caregiver support group, the local chapter of the Alzheimer's Association, family, friends, and faith groups. You may want to join a support group of Alzheimer's disease caregivers. These groups meet in person or online to share experiences and tips and give each other support. Ask your doctor, check online, or contact the local chapter of the Alzheimer's Association. Mental health professionals and social workers help you deal with any stress you may be feeling. They help you understand feelings, such as anger, sadness, or feeling out of control. They can also help you make plans for unexpected or sudden events. Mental health professionals charge by the hour. Medicare, Medicaid, and some private health insurance plans may cover some of these costs. Ask your health insurance plan which mental health counselors and services it covers. Then check with your doctor, local family service agencies, and community mental health agencies for referrals to counselors.

To learn where to get help in your community, contact

- Alzheimer's Disease Education and Referral (ADEAR) Center, 1-800-438-4380 or www.nia.nih.gov/alzheimers
- Alzheimer's Association, 1-800-272-3900 or www.alz.org
- Eldercare Locator, 1-800-677-1116 or www.eldercare.gov

You can also contact your local area agency on aging.

24. What are effective ways to ask for help?

Everyone needs help at times. However, many caregivers find it hard to ask for help. They may feel they should be able to do everything themselves, or that it's not all right to leave the person in their care with someone else. Or maybe they can't afford to pay someone to watch the person for an hour or two. Family members, friends, and community resources can help caregivers of people with Alzheimer's disease. Here are some tips about asking for help.

- It's okay to ask for help from family, friends, and others. You don't have to do everything yourself.
- Ask people to help out in specific ways, like making a meal, visiting the person, or taking the person out for a short time.
- Call for help from home health care or adult day care services when needed.
- Use national and local resources to find out how to pay for some of this help.

To learn where to get help in your community, contact

- The Alzheimer's Disease Education and Referral (ADEAR) Center, 1-800-438-4380 or www.nia.nih.gov/alzheimers
- The Alzheimer's Association, 1-800-272-3900 or www.alz.org
- The Eldercare Locator, 1-800-677-1116 or www.eldercare.gov.

You can also contact your local area agency on aging.

25. If you need to take a break or go away on vacation, what services are available to care for the person with Alzheimer's?

Respite services provide short stays, from a few days to a few weeks, in a nursing home or other place for the person with Alzheimer's disease. This care allows you to get a break or go on a vacation.

Respite services charge by the number of days or weeks that services are provided. Medicare or Medicaid may cover the cost of up to 5 days in a row of respite care in an inpatient facility. Most private insurance plans do not cover these costs. To find respite services in your community, visit the National Respite Locator Service at www.respitelocator.org.

26. If you are feeling burned out from caregiving, what can you do?

Caring for a person with Alzheimer's takes a lot of time and effort. Sometimes, you may feel discouraged, sad, lonely, frustrated, confused, or angry. These feelings are normal. Here are some things you can say to yourself that might help you feel better.

- I'm doing the best I can.
- What I'm doing would be hard for anyone.
- I'm not perfect, and that's okay.
- I can't control some things that happen.
- Sometimes, I just need to do what works for right now.

- I will try to get help from a counselor if caregiving becomes too much for me.

You may want to join a support group of Alzheimer's disease caregivers. These groups meet in person or online to share experiences and tips and give each other support. Ask your doctor, check online, or contact the local chapter of the Alzheimer's Association.

Some caregivers find that going to a church, temple, or mosque helps them cope with the daily demands placed on them. For others, simply having a sense that larger forces are at work in the world helps them find a sense of balance and peace.

Other MedicalCenter.com Publications

The Key Facts on Arthritis

The Key Facts on Breast Cancer

The Key Facts on Medicare

The Key Facts on Alzheimer's Disease

All Titles Can Be Found at

www.Amazon.com

www.MedicalCenter.com

CPSIA information can be obtained at www.ICGtesting.com
Printed in the USA
BVOW06s1052300516

449993BV00012B/72/P